Smoothies for Beginners

A Smoothie Recipe Book for Healthy Living

By

Dermot Farrell

Contents

Introduction – Smoothies for Health

Smoothies have many benefits to health, which includes:

•   Acting as a nutritional top up: The ultimate natural supplementation program for busy people, or people who do not have a voracious appetite.

•   Ill health preventative :   Because vegetables and fruits contain so many nutrients and antioxidants, they help to build up the immune system and ward off ill health.

•   Raw is gold :   Because juicing means that we are eating raw (uncooked) fruits and vegetables, it also means that we are receiving the full benefit of the nutrients, with no diminution , which occurs during the cooking process.

•   Cure – all :   Once again because of the many nutrients and antioxidants which they possess, fruits and vegetables, when juiced can often help to recover from ill health. Partly, because they are concentrated nutritional supplements (for example you couldn't eat 10 carrots, but you could drink them), and also because of the many unique elements such as flavonoids, anti-oxidants, phytonutrients, to mention but a few.

•   Unique Benefits: Such as the anti-inflammatory properties of some plants and the anti-histamine effects of others; while still other plants have either a cleansing effect on the liver or a balancing effect on the stomach, for instance.

These are just a quick overview of the more famous health boosting effects of juicing vegetables and fruits.

But what about smoothies, are they the same or do they possess more or less health giving benefits?

In a nutshell smoothies are actually healthier. Because the difference between taking a juice and taking a smoothy is that we filter out the sediment when we take a juice, whereas with a smooth we drink the entire concoction.

Now the sediment possesses both nutrients and fibre, both of which are good for health. Nutrients help to make us healthier and fibre both cleanses the intestinal system, as well as aiding blood sugar regulation and it also helps to create a feeling of satiation, whereby we don't want to eat more food, which is good for dieting.

Another benefit of smoothies, is that a fruit smooth will tend to be really delicious, because you are taking something which tastes great, like strawberries, for instance, and eating them whole, rather than just their juice, which again is great.

Why then opt for juices?

Where juices come in handy, is in their ease of consumption. A strawberry smoothie will be delicious, but how about a kale smoothie? I think not.

Simply put, the majority of fruits and vegetables either taste bad or they are simply difficult to ingest, in smoothie format, as they tend to possess grainy sticky sediment, which doesn't go down well.

Furthermore, for some people, particularly the sick and the weak, ingesting a fibrous smoothie may be too much work to handle. A person with intestinal or stomach issues, a cancer patient or a person coming of off a long fast may find it overwhelming to attempt to digest a smoothie. Better that they start with a juice, which will be far less taxing on their system.

Also, for people on a diet, the calories contained in a juice can basically be ignored because they are:

A). Very low

B). The body is probably going to expend a similar amount of energy in absorbing them.

However, smoothness while delicious, can easily be very high in calories, especially when you start combining fruits like bananas with milk, for example. This tastes great and is a wonderful post workout supercharger, but alas it's not good for those who are on a diet!

Obviously then our choices of smoothies are less, but have no fear the smoothies contained in this book are both tasty and healthy and go down easily!

Chapter One – Smoothies for Anxiety

Banana Berry De Luxe

INGREDIENTS:

- 3 bananas
- ½ cup of frozen berries
- 2 peaches
- Handful of spinach
- 1 cup of natural yoghurt

Procedure:

1. Place the fruit and vegetables into a blender.

2. Blend until smooth.

3. Add some extra natural yoghurt if you want to make it more liquidy.

4. Add sugar or honey if you want to make sweeter.

BENEFITS:

Bananas: Contain tryptophan (which helps to boost serotonin (the feel good neurotransmitter) levels in the brain). Also they are high in vitamin B, which aids brain function.

Blueberries: Are high in antioxidants and vitamin C, and are generally good for health, and possess a good taste.

Peaches: Possess natural sedative properties.

Spinach: Is high in magnesium, which helps to regulate cortisol levels in the body. Since cortisol is a stress hormone (which is released during times of stress) it helps when we have to deal with trauma or face survival decisions, however it is destructive for health in the long-term. So regulating it, is a good way to help reduce anxiety, as many of us suffer from inordinately high cortisol levels, on a daily basis.

Natural Yoghurt: Tastes great and is a good base of the smoothly. Also it is full of healthy bacteria, which help to both clean out and regulate our intestines. Since many people suffer from constipation, which also worsens their anxiety levels, so natural yoghurt will be a help to them.

Coco Boost

Ingredients:

- 3 Bananas

- ½ a pineapple

- Half a cup of coconut powder

- Either 500ml of cold milk or 500ml of natural yoghurt or 1 cup of ice cubes and 300 ml of cold water.

Procedure:

1. Place the fruit into a blender.

2. Blend until smooth.

3. Add some extra natural yoghurt in if you want to make it more liquidy.

4. Add sugar or honey if you want to make sweeter.

Benefits:

Bananas: Contain tryptophan (which helps to boost serotonin (the feel good neurotransmitter) levels in the brain). Also they are high in vitamin B, which aids brain function.

Pineapples: Are high in B vitamins and are known for their mental relaxation properties.

Spinach: Is high in magnesium, which helps to regulate cortisol levels in the body. Since cortisol is a stress hormone (which is released during times of stress) it helps when we have to deal with trauma or face survival decisions, however it is destructive for health in the long-term. So regulating it, is a good way to help reduce anxiety, as many of us suffer from inordinately high cortisol levels, on a daily basis.

Coconuts: Coconuts add taste and also possess many health general health benefits, which includes, immunity boosting, heart health protection and protection against brain disorders, such as Alzheimer's.

Avocado Twist

Ingredients:

- 3 avocadoes
- A handful of mint leaves
- 1 pineapple
- Either 500ml of cold milk or 500ml of natural yoghurt or 1 cup of ice cubes and 300 ml of cold water.

Procedure:

1.   Place the fruit and vegetables into a blender.

2.   Blend until smooth.

3.   Add some extra natural yoghurt in if you want to make it more liquidy.

4.   Add sugar or honey if you want to make sweeter.

Benefits:

Avocadoes: Are high in potassium and vitamin B. They are well known for their ability to reduce blood pressure and to bring about a relaxed state.

Mint: Is renowned for its relaxing properties.

Pineapples: Are high in B vitamins and are known for their mental relaxation properties.

Chapter Two – Smoothies for Allergies

Grapple The Apple

Ingredients:

- 4 large apples

- 2 cups of grapes (preferably red or black)

- 3 carrots

- 1 cup of ice cubes and 300ml of cold water or 500lm of cold milk or 500ml of natural yoghurt

Procedure:

1. Place the fruit and vegetables into a blender.

2. Blend until smooth.

3. Add some extra natural yoghurt in if you want to make it more liquidy.

4. Add sugar or honey if you want to make sweeter.

Benefits:

Apples: Apples are high in Quercetin, which is a natural anti-histamine.

Grapes: Grapes are high in Quercetin, which is a natural anti-histamine.

Carrots: Contain beta-carotene, which is good for allergies.

Peach Delight!

Ingredients:

- 3 Peaches
- 3 oranges
- 3 bananas
- 1 cup of ice cubes and 300ml of cold water or 500lm of cold milk or 500ml of natural yoghurt

Procedure:

1. Place the fruit into a blender.

2. Blend until smooth.

3. Add some extra natural yoghurt in if you want to make it more liquid.

4. Add sugar or honey if you want to make sweeter.

Benefits:

Peaches: Are high in Quercetin, which is natural anti-histamine.

Oranges: Are high in vitamin C, which reduces inflammation which goes along with allergic conditions.

Bananas: Brings relief to persons who suffer with skin rashes, asthmatic allergic reactions and digestive allergic responses. Apart from that they are generally nutritious and they taste great. Although in some cases bananas should be avoided. Bananas increase phlegm, in the body, which is bad news for anyone who suffers with rhinitis or sinusitis. If taken occasionally they are usually fine, but if taken repeatedly (as in several a day) often they worsen these symptoms.,

Extreme Fruit Twist

Ingredients:

- 1 knob of garlic.
- 1 knob of ginger
- 2 cups of berries(either strawberries, blue berries or acai berries)
- 3 peaches
- 1 cup of ice cubes and 300ml of cold water or 500lm of cold milk or 500ml of natural yoghurt

Procedure:

1.   Place the fruit and vegetables into a blender.

2.   Blend until smooth.

3.   Add some extra natural yoghurt in if you want to make it more liquid.

4.   Add sugar or honey if you want to make sweeter.

Benefits:

Garlic: Boosts the immune system, which helps to fend of allergies.

Ginger: Ginger is a natural anti-histamine.

Berries: Are high in Quercetin, which is a natural anti-histamine.

Peaches: Are high in Quercetin, which is a natural anti-histamine.

Chapter Three – Cold & Flu

Orange Coconut Ginger Twist

Ingredients:

- 3 Oranges
- 1 cup of coconut powder and or 50ml of coconut oil and or 100ml of coconut water
- 3 pieces of ginger
- 1 cup of ice cubes and 300ml of cold water or 500lm of cold milk or 500ml of natural yoghurt

Procedure:

1. Place the fruit and vegetables into a blender.

2. Blend until smooth.

3. Add some extra natural yoghurt in if you want to make it more liquidy.

4. Add sugar or honey if you want to make sweeter.

Benefits:

Oranges: Are high in vitamin C, which boosts the immune system.

Coconuts: Are really healthy. Coconut powder is full of anti-bacterial, anti-fungal and anti-viral properties. Coconut water is high in electrolytes, which rehydrates the body, which is useful if you have a fever. Coconut oil contains 'lauric acid' which is full of anti-bacterial, antifungal and antiviral properties.

Ginger: Has strong anti-bacterial properties. It is also an anti-inflammatory, which helps to reduce painful swelling.

Garlic Coconut Berry Blaster

Ingredients:

- 1 cup of coconut powder and or 50ml of coconut oil and or 100ml of coconut water
- 1 cup of berries (blue berries, strawberries or any kind of berry)
- 3 oranges
- 1 large lemon
- 3 cloves of ginger
- 5 cloves of garlic
- 1 cup of ice cubes and 300ml of cold water or 500ml of cold milk or 500ml of natural yoghurt

Procedure:

1. Place the fruit and vegetables into a blender.

2. Blend until smooth.

3. Add some extra natural yoghurt in if you want to make it more liquid.

4. Add sugar or honey if you want to make sweeter.

Benefits:

Coconuts: Are really healthy. Coconut powder is full of anti-bacterial, anti-fungal and anti-viral properties. Coconut water is high in electrolytes, which rehydrates the body, which is useful if you have a fever. Coconut oil contains 'lauric acid' which is full of anti-bacterial, antifungal and antiviral properties.

Oranges: Are high in vitamin C, which boosts the immune system.

Berries: Boost the immune system.

Lemons: Are high in vitamin C, which boost the immune system.

Ginger: Has strong anti-bacterial properties. It is also an anti-inflammatory, which helps to reduce painful swelling.

Garlic: Has strong anti-bacterial properties, and has been proven to reduce the duration of the common cold.

Berry Fruit Twist

Ingredients:

- 1 cup of berries
- 3 kiwis
- 2 avocadoes
- 3 apples
- 1 cup of ice cubes and 300ml of cold water or 500ml of cold milk or 500ml of natural yoghurt

Procedure:

1. Place the fruit into a blender.
2. Blend until smooth.
3. Add some extra natural yoghurt in if you want to make it more liquidy.
4. Add sugar or honey if you want to make sweeter.

Benefits:

Berries: Boost the immune system.

Kiwis: Are high in vitamin C which boosts the immune system.

Avocados: Are high in vitamin C, which boosts the immune system.

Apples: Are high in vitamin C, which boosts the immune system.

Chapter Four – Headache

Pineapple Burst

Ingredients:

- 250ml of coconut water
- 1 pineapple
- 1 lemon
- 2 cucumbers
- 1 piece of ginger
- 1 cup of kale
- 1 cup of ice cubes and 300ml of cold water or 500ml of cold milk or 500ml of natural yoghurt

Procedure:

1. Place the fruit and vegetables into a blender.

2. Blend until smooth.

3. Add some extra natural yoghurt in if you want to make it more liquidy.

4. Add sugar or honey if you want to make sweeter.

Benefits:

Lemons: Relax the body, plus they are hydrating and help to balance out pH Levels in the body.

Ginger: Has been noted to have a positive effect on headaches. Why exactly is as yet unknown. The positive effect is probably due to its many health enhancing properties.

Pineapple: Contains the enzyme bromelain, which are natural pain reliever and anti- inflammatory.

Cucumbers: Are hydrating, which is helpful as often headaches are made more intense due to dehydration.

Kale: Is quite famous for its headache relieving benefits, although we areas yet uncertain why exactly kale is such a great headache relieve go to food.

Rehydrate Your Melon!

Ingredients:

- 1 cup of kale
- ¼ of a watermelon
- 3 cucumbers
- 1 pineapple
- 1 celery stalk
- 1 large lemon
- 250ml of coconut water
- 1 clove of garlic
- 1 cup of ice cubes and 300ml of cold water or 500ml of cold milk or 500ml of natural yoghurt

Procedure:

1.   Place the fruit and vegetables into a blender.
2.   Blend until smooth.
3.   Add some extra natural yoghurt in if you want to make it more liquidy.
4.   Add sugar or honey if you want to make sweeter.

Benefits:

Lemons: Relax the body, plus they are hydrating and help to balance out ph. Levels.

Ginger: Has been noted to have a positive effect on headaches. Why exactly is as yet unknown. The positive effect is probably due to its many health enhancing properties.

Pineapple: Contains the enzyme bromelain, which are natural pain relievers and anti- inflammatories.

Cucumbers: Are hydrating, which is helpful as often headaches are made more intense due to dehydration.

Kale: Is quite famous for its headache relieving benefits, although we areas yet uncertain why exactly kale is such a great headache relieve go to food.

Celery: Is high on luteolin, an anti-inflammatory flavonoid, which helps to reduce headaches.

WTERMELON: Is extremely hydrating, and is high in natural sugars, which can be quite invigorating.

Coconut water: Is high in electrolytes, which help to rehydrate and rebalance the body during bouts of fever. Also many headaches occur due to dehydration and from loss of salts (electrolytes), so they help to rebalance this.

This is Bananas!

Ingredients:

- 250ml of coconut water
- 5 bananas
- 1 cup of raspberries
- 2 avocados

Procedure:

1. Place the fruit into a blender.
2. Blend until smooth.
3. Add some extra natural yoghurt in if you want to make it more liquid.
4. Add sugar or honey if you want to make sweeter.

Benefits:

Coconut water is high in electrolytes which help to rehydrate and rebalance the body during bouts of fever. Also many headaches occur due to dehydration and a loss of salts (electrolytes), so they help to rebalance this.

Bananas: Are high in vitamin B, which boosts serotonin levels, which is de-stressing and so can help to relieve headaches.

Strawberries/Blueberries/Raspberries: Are all high on naturally occurring aspirin, which reliefs the symptoms of headache.

Chapter Five – Stomach

Banana Relief

Ingredients:

- 3 bananas
- 2 avocados
- 1 cup of aloe vera gel or liquid
- 2tbsp's of honey
- 1 cup of ice cubes and 300ml of cold water or 500ml of cold milk or 500ml of natural yoghurt

Procedure:

1. Place the fruit and aloe Vera oil into a blender.

2. Blend until smooth.

3. Add some extra natural yoghurt in if you want to make it more liquid.

4. Add sugar or honey if you want to make sweeter.

Benefits:

Bananas: Contain pectin, which helps with bowel movements. Often stomach aches result from blocked intestines which results in the intestines becoming bigger, which then presses (painfully) against the stomach.

Avocados: Reduce inflammation in the stomach lining.

Aloe Vera: Improves digestive functioning thus relieving stomach ache.

Honey: Reduces inflammation of the oesophagus and stomach lining and also it has a soothing effect which helps both with stomach ache and with acid reflux.

Papaya Yoghurt Twist

Ingredients:

- 1 papaya
- 1 knob of ginger
- 3 tbsp. of honey
- 1 cup of ice cubes and 300ml of cold water or 500ml of cold milk or 500ml of natural yoghurt

Procedure:

1. Place the fruit and ginger and cold water/milk/natural yoghurt into a blender.

2. Blend until smooth.

3. Add some extra natural yoghurt in if you want to make it more liquid.

4. Add sugar or honey if you want to make sweeter.

Benefits:

Papaya: Helps to settle the stomach

Ginger: Improves the digestive system and also helps out with nausea.

Natural Yoghurt: Is a great probiotic and helps to fill the stomach with friendly bacteria, which aid in digestion. Natural yoghurt is also a base and helps to reduce acidity in the stomach.

Honey: Reduces inflammation of the oesophagus and stomach lining and also it has a soothing effect which helps both with stomach ache and with acid reflux.

"Wow I Love This Sweet Tasting Fruit Yoghurt Mix!"

Ingredients:

- 3 cups of strawberries
- 5 medium sized peaches
- 1000ml of natural yoghurt

Procedure:

1. Place the fruit and natural yoghurt into a blender.

2. Blend until smooth.

3. Add some extra natural yoghurt or milk in if you want to make it more liquid.

4. Add sugar or honey if you want to make sweeter.

Benefits:

Strawberries: Reduce inflammation of the stomach lining thus relieving gastritis,

Peaches: Boost the digestive process, and they also taste really good!

Honey: Reduces inflammation of the oesophagus and stomach lining and also it has a soothing effect which helps both with stomach ache and with acid reflux.

Chapter Six – Nausea

Triple Reliever

Ingredients:

- 3 pears
- 3 apples
- 3 carrots
- 1 cup of ice cubes and 300ml of cold water or 500lm of cold milk or 500ml of natural yoghurt

Procedure:

1. Place the fruit, natural yoghurt or milk or cold water into a blender.

2. Blend until smooth.

3. Add some extra natural yoghurt in if you want to make it more liquid.

4. Add sugar or honey if you want to make sweeter.

Benefits:

Pears: Help to absorb excess acid thus reducing acid reflux.

Apples: Help to settle the stomach.

Carrots: Settle the stomach.

Banana Papaya Boost

Ingredients:

- 6 bananas
- 1 papaya
- A handful of mint leaves
- 1 cup of ice cubes and 300ml of cold water or 500ml of cold milk or 500ml of natural yoghurt

Procedure:

1. Place the fruit, natural yoghurt and cold water into a blender.

2. Blend until smooth.

3. Add some extra natural yoghurt in if you want to make it more liquid.

4. Add sugar or honey if you want to make sweeter.

Benefits:

Bananas: Settle the stomach. Also they are high in potassium, which is useful if you are dehydrated after vomiting, as electrolytes are lost every time we vomit. For anyone who is vomiting, they should take either electrolytes, in water solution, or take in something like a banana shake or banana smoothie.

Papaya: Settles the stomach

Mint: Settles the stomach.

The Hydra King

Ingredients:

- Half a watermelon
- 5 bananas
- 1 cup(250ml-1/2 pint) of coconut water
- 500ml of natural yoghurt

Procedure:

1. Place the fruit, natural yoghurt and cold water into a blender.

2. Blend until smooth.

3. Add some extra natural yoghurt in if you want to make it more liquid.

4. Add sugar or honey if you want to make sweeter.

Benefits:

Watermelon: Is very high in water which rehydrates. Also, it is high in potassium which make up for lost electrolytes (lost in vomiting) and vitamin C (which boosts the immune system and fights infection).

Bananas: Settle the stomach. Also they are high in potassium, which is useful if you are dehydrated after vomiting, as electrolytes are lost every time we vomit. For anyone who is vomiting they should take either electrolyte, in water solution, or take in something like a banana shake or banana smoothie.

Coconut Water: Is full of electrolytes and also essential minerals such as potassium, calcium, sodium and phosphorous and magnesium.

Chapter Seven – Acne and Skin

Berry Coco Mix

Ingredients:

- 1 cup of berries (ideally blueberries but strawberries or raspberries will also do).
- 250 ml (1/2 pint) of coconut water
- 1 avocado
- 1tbsp of raw cacao powder (coco will do if you cannot get cacao powder)
- 1 cup of ice cubes and 300ml of cold water or 500ml of cold milk or 500ml of natural yoghurt

Procedure:

1. Place the fruit, cacao powder, ginger and coconut water and either water , milk or yoghurt into a blender.

2. Blend until smooth.

3. Add some extra natural yoghurt in if you want to make it more liquid.

4. Add sugar or honey if you want to make sweeter.

Benefits:

Berries: Are good for skin quality.

Avocado: Is full of antioxidants which help to detox the skin

Cocoa Powder: Is full of anti-oxidants which help to detox the skin.

Coconut Milk: Helps to hydrate the skin.

Almond Fruit Twist

Ingredients:

- 3 bananas
- 1 cup of almonds (they should be soaked in water overnight so as to gain the maximum benefit from them)
- 1 tbsp. of flax seeds
- 1 apple
- 2 pears
- 1 cup of ice cubes and 300ml of cold water or 500ml of cold milk or 500ml of natural yoghurt

Procedure:

1. Place the fruit, natural yoghurt or cold water into a blender.

2. Blend until smooth.

3. Add some extra natural yoghurt in if you want to make it more liquid.

4. Add sugar or honey if you want to make sweeter.

Benefits:

Bananas: Are high in vitamin C and vitamin B6, which help to make skin elastic.

Almonds: Almonds (when soaked) help to rebuild damaged skin cells.

Apples: Are high in copper, vitamin C and potassium, all of which help to nourish the skin. Furthermore, they are high in antioxidants, which help to clear out fungal and bacterial infections from the skin.

Pears: Help to reduce acne. Also they are a cooling fruit. Skin conditions like acne and psoriasis, for example, always results in hot prickly skin. Eating pears will help to reduce the sting in these conditions.

Flax Seeds: Are high in omega 3 oil which helps to rebuild skin cells. Also they are high in Lignin's, which help to reduce DHT in the body, which in turn helps to rejuvenate the skin, in the case of acne.

Super Fruit Yoghurt Smoothie

Ingredients:

- 3 mangos
- 3 oranges
- 3 pears
- 1 cup of ice cubes and 300ml of cold water or 500ml of cold milk or 500ml of natural yoghurt

Procedure:

1. Place the fruit, natural yoghurt or cold water into a blender.

2. Blend until smooth.

3. Add some extra natural yoghurt in if you want to make it more liquid.

4. Add sugar or honey if you want to make sweeter.

Benefits:

Mangos: Are high in vitamins B6, C and E, all of which have skin nurturing qualities.

Oranges: Are high in vitamin C which is good for skin.

Pears: Help to reduce acne. Also they are a cooling fruit. Skin conditions like acne and psoriasis, for example, always results in hot prickly sin. Eating pears will help to reduce the sting of these conditions.

Natural yoghurt: Is high on antioxidants which help skin quality.

Chapter Eight – Arthritis

Pineapple Crush

Ingredients:

- 1 pineapple
- 3 oranges
- 1 cup of ice cubes and 300ml of cold water or 500ml of cold milk or 500ml of natural yoghurt

Procedure:

1. Place the fruit, natural yoghurt or cold water into a blender.
2. Add honey or sugar for sweetness if needed.
3. Blend and serve

Benefits:

Pineapples: Are high in bromelain, which reduces arthritic pain.

Oranges: Are high in vitamin C, which helps to reduce inflammation and is very helpful at reducing symptoms of gout.

Berry Blast

Ingredients:

- 2 apples
- 2 cups of grapes
- 3 cups of berries (blueberries, strawberries or raspberries)
- 1 cup of ice cubes and 300ml of cold water or 500ml of cold milk or 500ml of natural yoghurt.

Procedure:

1. Place the fruit, natural yoghurt or cold water into a blender.
2. Add honey or sugar for sweetness if needed.
3. Blend and serve.

Benefits:

Berries, grapes and apples are all high in quercetin, and quercetin makes a big impact in reducing inflammation.

Yummy Fruit Blast

Ingredients:

- 3 medium sized guava
- 3 medium sized kiwi fruits
- 3 oranges

- 1 cup of ice cubes and 300ml of cold water or 500ml of cold milk or 500ml of natural yoghurt

Procedure:

1. Place the fruit, natural yoghurt or cold water into a blender.
2. Add honey or sugar for sweetness if needed.
3. Blend and serve.

Benefits:

Guava: Is well known for its anti-inflammatory properties

Kiwis and Oranges: Are high in vitamin C, which is good for arthritis.

Chapter Nine – High Blood Pressure

Blueberry Banana Twist

Ingredients:

- 3 cups of blueberries
- 3 bananas
- 500ml of natural yoghurt

Procedure:

1. Place the fruit, natural yoghurt or cold water into a blender.
2. Add honey or sugar to sweeten if necessary.
3. Blend and serve,

Benefits:

Blueberries: Have been noted for its ability to substantially reduce blood pressure levels. Why exactly, we're not sure yet, but in clinical tests a cup serving will reduce blood pressure levels by about 5%.

Bananas: May or may not work. Potassium has an important part to play in blood pressure regulations. If your body is lacking potassium, then bananas will really help, otherwise it won't help, but it will still taste good!

Tangy Fruit Twist

Ingredients:

- 3 knobs of garlic
- 1 knobs of ginger
- 3 avocados
- 3 bananas
- 1 cup of ice cubes and 300ml of cold water or 500ml of cold milk or 500ml of natural yoghurt.

Procedure:

1. Peel the garlic and the ginger and slice them into little bits.
2. Add in the avocados, bananas and either yoghurt or water.
3. Blend and serve.

Benefits:

Garlic and Ginger: Produce a noted effect on lowering blood pressure levels.

Bananas: May or may not work. Potassium has an important part to play in blood pressure regulations IF your body is lacking potassium then bananas will really help, otherwise it won't help, but it will still taste good!

Avocados: Like bananas are high in potassium which may lower blood pressure levels in some cases. Also, they are extremely good for heart health.

Fruit Explosion!!!

Ingredients:

- 3 cups of strawberries
- 3 bananas
- 3 kiwis
- 3 avocados
- 1 cup of ice cubes and 300ml of cold water or 500ml of cold milk or 500ml of natural yoghurt.

Procedure:

1. Place the fruit, natural yoghurt or cold water into a blender.
2. Blend and serve

Benefits:

Bananas: May or may not work. Potassium has an important part to play in blood pressure regulations IF your body is lacking potassium then bananas will really help, otherwise it won't help, but it will still taste good!

Avocados: Like bananas are high in potassium which may lower blood pressure levels in some cases. Also, they are extremely good for heart health.

Berries: Have been demonstrated in laboratory conditions to have a substantial effect on blood pressure reduction

Chapter Ten – Diabetes

Green Blast

Ingredients:

- 1 handful of spinach
- 3 cucumbers
- 2 celery stalks
- 3 cinnamon rolls
- 3 knobs of ginger
- 500 ml of water

Procedure:

1. Place the vegetables and water into a blender.
2. Blend and serve

Benefits:

Spinach Is high in magnesium which helps diabetics to balance their sugar levels.

Cucumbers Are hydrating, which helps diabetics and also it is high in fibre which helps to reduce blood sugar levels.

Celery Is high in vitamin k, which reduces inflammation and increases insulin sensitivity, which in turn benefits blood sugar control.

Cinnamon   Is very powerful when it comes to reducing blood sugar levels. Why cinnamon works so effectively, is still vague, but certainly in clinical trials it has worked very effectively.

Ginger: Is a general tonic, and has been proven as a diabetic treatment which reduces blood glucose levels in the blood.

Green Berry Blast

Ingredients:

- 1 handful of kale
- 3 aloe Vera leafs
- 2 tsp. of cardamom seeds
- 3 cups of berries (strawberry, raspberry or blueberries)
- 500 ml almond milk

Procedure:

1. Place the vegetables, fruits and seed and almond water into a blender.
2. Blend and serve.

Benefits:

Kale: Is high in vitamins A and K and potassium, all of which helps to reduce symptoms of diabetes.

Aloe Vera: Helps to regulate sugar levels

Cardamom Seeds: Have been demonstrated to lower blood sugar levels.

Berries: Are high in fibre and vitamin C and antioxidants, which help diabetics.

Almond Milk: Is high in magnesium, manganese, potassium and selenium, all of which help to reduce diabetic symptoms.

Fruit Lassi

Ingredients:

- 3 cups of strawberries
- 3 bananas
- 1 papaya
- 500 ml of natural yoghurt

Procedure:

1. Mix the fruits in with the yoghurt.
2. Add cold water if you wish to dilute.
3. Blend and serve.

Benefits:

This smoothy is a treat for diabetics. Although it's absolutely delicious and sweet in taste, its actual good for your health. Strawberries are good for diabetes and are low in sugar. Although bananas are high in carbohydrates, they are slow releasing, and bananas are high in potassium, which is good for diabetics. Papaya is an amazing fruit, which is very low on sugar and which is high in vitamins, fibre and antioxidants. Also, natural yoghurt is high in probiotics and protein while been low in carbs.

Chapter Eleven – Menopause

Nutty Green Berry Mix

Ingredients:

- 1 handful of kale
- 1 handful of spinach
- 1 knob of garlic
- 1 knob of ginger
- 3 cups of berries(strawberry, raspberry or blueberries)
- 50 grams of almonds
- 500 ml of natural yoghurt or 500 ml of milk

Procedure:

1. Add the vegetables, fruit and milk into a blender.
2. Blend and drink.

Benefits:

Kale: Is high in vitamins K and E, which is beneficial, as is magnesium, which helps to reduce hot flashes.

Spinach: Like kale is high in magnesium, which is good for hot flashes.

Spinach and kale: Are nutrient dense, with the sheer total percentage of nutrients helping to rebalance menopausal symptoms on various levels.

Garlic and Ginger: Are both very powerful tonics, which can recharge the body's energy levels and can also help to make the menopause far gentler.

Almonds: Are high vitamin B12, zinc and iron. Also, almonds are particularly good at reducing anxiety symptoms.

Beanny Mix

Ingredients:

- 1 handful of soy beans
- 1 handful of sunflower seeds
- 1 knob of garlic
- 1 knob of ginger
- 3 kiwis
- 500 ml of almond milk

Procedure:

1. Grind the various seeds.
2. Then miss in the seeds with the garlic and ginger, kiwis and almond milk.
3. Blend and serve.

Benefits:

Soybeans: Contain phytoestrogens, which boost estrogen levels in the body, thus reducing the intensity of menopausal symptoms.

Sunflower: Seeds are high in vitamin E, which helps to reduce hot flushes.

Garlic and Ginger: Are both very powerful tonics, which can recharge the body's energy levels and can also help to make the menopause far gentler.

Almonds: Are high vitamin B12, zinc and iron. Also, almonds are particularly good at reducing anxiety symptoms.

Kiwis: Are high in vitamins C which help to reduce hot flushes.

Fruit & Nut Lassi/Milkshake

Ingredients:

- 3 cups of berries (blueberries, strawberries, raspberries)
- 3 avocados
- 3 kiwis
- 3 handfuls of almonds
- 500 ml of natural yoghurt or milk

Procedure:

1. Mix the fruits, almonds and yoghurt/milk.
2. Add honey or sugar to sweeten as necessary.
3. Blend and serve.

Benefits:

Berries: Help to reduced hot flushes.

Avocados: The plant sterols in avocados boost oestrogen and progesterone levels, which reduce menopausal symptoms.

Kiwis: Are high in vitamin C which helps to reduce hot flushes.

Almonds: Are high vitamin B12, zinc and iron. Also, almonds are particularly good at reducing anxiety symptoms.